CYCLIC DIETING

Burn Fat and Lose Weight

By Jasmin Brooks

Introduction

Are you tired of diets that restrict your favorite foods and leave you feeling drained? Discover a new, science-backed approach to eating that boosts metabolism, enhances energy, and helps you reach your health and fitness goals—without the constant cycle of deprivation. In *Cyclic Dieting: Burn Fat and Lose Weight*, you'll learn how to harness the benefits of carb cycling and meal timing to transform your body and mind.

Overview of Cyclic Dieting and Its Benefits

Cyclic nutrition, often referred to as carb cycling or macro cycling, is a dietary approach designed to optimize metabolic health, enhance energy levels, and support specific fitness goals like weight loss, muscle growth, and athletic performance. Unlike many restrictive diets, cyclic nutrition doesn't rely on extreme calorie reduction or cutting out entire food groups; instead, it strategically varies macronutrient intake over time. This approach helps the body efficiently use nutrients, boosts energy and recovery, and reduces common diet-related frustrations such as plateaus and burnout.

At its core, cyclic nutrition operates on the principle of fluctuating carbohydrate intake, typically in a planned cycle, while keeping protein and fat intake steady or varied according to the individual's needs. The cycle might involve alternating between high-carbohydrate, low-carbohydrate, and balanced-macronutrient days, adapting these levels based on activity level and specific body goals.

Key benefits of cyclic nutrition include:

- **Efficient fat burning**: Periodic low-carb days encourage the body to use stored fat for energy.

- **Improved energy and performance**: High-carb days replenish glycogen stores, boosting physical and mental energy.

- **Hormone balance**: Alternating carbohydrate intake supports leptin, insulin, and other hormones, helping the body respond well to nutrient intake and avoid adapting too fully to a single diet.

- **Sustainable lifestyle**: Cyclic nutrition provides dietary flexibility, making it easier to sustain over time than diets that are more rigid or exclusionary.

Brief History of Cyclic Eating in Fitness and Wellness

The concept of cyclic eating has roots in various fitness and wellness practices, including bodybuilding, endurance sports, and traditional health systems. Early iterations of carb cycling began in bodybuilding communities, where athletes needed a reliable method to reduce body fat while preserving muscle mass. Bodybuilders noticed that alternating high- and low-carbohydrate days helped them achieve a lean and toned appearance without sacrificing muscle—a significant breakthrough for athletes who trained intensively.

Over time, this cyclic approach gained traction beyond bodybuilding and became popular among endurance athletes, who found that periodic high-carb days supported glycogen replenishment, enhancing stamina and endurance. Similarly, the wellness community recognized that cyclic eating not only supported physical performance but also metabolic and hormonal health, making it a versatile approach adaptable for individuals at various fitness levels and life stages.

Purpose and Scope of the Book

The purpose of this book is to offer a comprehensive guide to cyclic nutrition, breaking down its principles and applications in a way that is accessible, actionable, and sustainable for readers of all backgrounds. Whether the goal is weight loss, muscle gain, or simply a healthier and more balanced relationship with food, cyclic nutrition provides a flexible framework that can be customized to suit individual preferences and lifestyles.

In addition to providing the foundational science behind cyclic dieting, this book will walk readers through the process of setting goals, calculating nutritional needs, and implementing effective cycles tailored to their personal objectives. Practical examples, meal plans, and recipes will make it easy to put theory into practice, while insights into common challenges and troubleshooting tips will equip readers to stay motivated and adapt their approach as they progress.

The scope of the book includes:

- A **deep dive into macronutrients** and their role in cyclic nutrition
- **Practical guidelines** for structuring high-carb, low-carb, and balanced days
- **Step-by-step instructions** for planning cycles based on individual goals
- **Lifestyle considerations** including exercise, sleep, and stress management
- **Advanced cyclic nutrition techniques** for those seeking tailored approaches
- **Sample meal plans, recipes, and food lists** to simplify meal planning

---

Who Can Benefit from Cyclic Dieting?

Cyclic nutrition is a versatile approach suitable for a wide range of individuals with varied fitness and wellness objectives. This section will clarify who stands to gain the most from adopting a cyclic nutrition plan and why it may be the ideal approach for anyone looking to take control of their health.

Target audiences for cyclic nutrition include:

1. **Individuals aiming for sustainable weight loss**: Cyclic nutrition's alternating high- and low-carb days encourage fat metabolism without causing energy crashes. This is a key benefit for those struggling with restrictive diets that often lead to yo-yo dieting.
2. **Athletes and active individuals**: For people who engage in regular training, especially high-intensity or endurance

exercises, cyclic nutrition supports energy needs and helps replenish glycogen stores, improving performance and recovery.

3. **People seeking muscle growth or body recomposition**: Those who want to gain muscle while minimizing fat gain can use cyclic nutrition to support anabolic processes on high-carb days and fat metabolism on low-carb days, creating a balanced approach to body composition.

4. **Individuals with hormonal concerns**: Cyclic nutrition supports hormonal health by balancing insulin, leptin, and other metabolic hormones, which can be disrupted in rigid diets. This approach can benefit those dealing with energy fluctuations, mood instability, or metabolic adaptations from prolonged dieting.

5. **Anyone looking to maintain a healthy, flexible diet**: Cyclic nutrition is a sustainable approach for people who want

to nourish their bodies without the rigidity of fad diets. It can be adapted to various lifestyles, including vegan, vegetarian, and gluten-free diets, making it highly customizable.

Content:

Chapter 1

Fundamentals of Cyclic Nutrition

What Are Macronutrients?

Macronutrients—proteins, fats, and carbohydrates—are the primary sources of energy and nutrients required by the body. Each macronutrient serves a specific function in energy production, tissue repair, and overall health, making them central to any nutrition plan.

- **Proteins**

    Proteins are essential for tissue repair, muscle growth, and immune function. Made up of amino acids, proteins play a vital role in building and maintaining lean muscle, which is crucial for metabolic health and recovery. When carbs are low, the body can also break down protein for energy, though this is not ideal. Therefore, adequate protein intake helps preserve muscle during low-carb days, ensuring the body has what it needs to repair and rebuild.

- **Fats**

Dietary fats are necessary for hormone production, brain health, and the absorption of fat-soluble vitamins (A, D, E, and K). Healthy fats, especially those found in foods like avocados, nuts, and olive oil, provide a slow-burning energy source, stabilizing blood sugar levels and curbing hunger on low-carb days. Additionally, fats play a key role in hormone regulation, particularly during low-carb periods when fat intake may increase to compensate for the reduction in carbs.

- **Carbohydrates**

Carbohydrates are the body's primary energy source and are broken down into glucose, fueling brain function and physical activity. For high-intensity training, carbs are particularly important as they replenish glycogen stores in muscles, which is necessary for sustained performance and recovery. In cyclic nutrition, strategically planned high-carb days ensure that glycogen levels are topped up, supporting energy and muscle function.

How Cyclic Nutrition Works

Cyclic nutrition revolves around the concept of alternating between high-carb and low-carb days to optimize metabolic function, support weight management, and enhance physical performance. This section will delve into the science and practical structure behind carb cycling, explaining why varying carbohydrate intake is both effective and sustainable.

- **High-Carbohydrate Days**

On high-carb days, individuals consume a larger proportion of carbohydrates to replenish muscle glycogen, enhance energy levels, and support metabolic health. These high-carb days are usually scheduled around intense workout days or when more physical or mental energy is required. High-carb days also positively influence hormones such as leptin, which helps regulate hunger and energy expenditure, making it easier to sustain the diet over time.

- **Low-Carbohydrate Days**

During low-carb days, the body is encouraged to use fat as its primary fuel source, making this approach beneficial for fat loss. By reducing carbohydrate intake periodically, insulin levels remain stable, and the body becomes more efficient at burning stored fat. Protein and fat intake remain stable, ensuring muscle preservation and satiety even when carbs are reduced.

- **The Science Behind Carb Cycling**

Carb cycling capitalizes on the body's ability to switch between burning carbohydrates and fats for fuel, which is known as metabolic flexibility. This metabolic adaptability is crucial for effective weight management and avoiding the energy crashes often associated with low-carb diets. Additionally, cyclic nutrition positively impacts hormone balance, particularly leptin and insulin, by preventing the body from adapting fully to either high- or low-carb conditions.

This alternating approach helps break through weight loss plateaus and supports muscle gain while avoiding the restrictive nature of many diets, making it easier to sustain long-term.

Cyclic Diet vs. Other Diets

In a space full of popular diets, cyclic nutrition offers unique advantages due to its flexibility and focus on balance. This section compares cyclic nutrition with other diets, emphasizing why it may be a more sustainable and results-oriented approach.

- **Comparison with Other Diets**
  - **Keto Diet**: The keto diet relies on extreme carb restriction, forcing the body into ketosis, where it burns fat for fuel. While effective for some, keto can be restrictive and challenging to maintain, especially for athletes needing quick energy.

Cyclic nutrition allows for both low- and high-carb days, providing the benefits of carb reduction without the strict limitations of keto.

- **Intermittent Fasting (IF)**: IF focuses on timing rather than macronutrient composition, typically involving eating windows and fasting periods. Although IF can be effective for weight loss, it doesn't address nutrient timing around exercise or individual macronutrient needs. Cyclic nutrition, by contrast, integrates macronutrient management and energy needs, allowing for greater flexibility in meal timing.
- **Calorie Restriction Diets**: Many traditional diets rely on simply cutting calories, often leading to short-term weight loss but potential

muscle loss and metabolic slowdown. Cyclic nutrition prioritizes nutrient timing and macronutrient manipulation, which can prevent the metabolic slowdowns and muscle loss that can occur with basic calorie restriction.

- **Advantages of Cyclic Nutrition**

Cyclic nutrition is designed to offer sustainability and flexibility by:

  - Supporting energy needs: High-carb days fuel intense workouts and cognitive function, while low-carb days enhance fat-burning potential.
  - Preserving muscle: The strategic use of carbs prevents the muscle breakdown that can occur in low-carb or low-calorie diets.

- Balancing hormones: Cyclic nutrition prevents the metabolic adaptation often seen in strict diets, supporting healthy levels of leptin, insulin, and other key hormones.
- Allowing flexibility: Unlike many rigid diets, cyclic nutrition offers room for personal preferences, training schedules, and lifestyle factors, making it easier to maintain over the long term.

Chapter 2

Setting Goals with Cyclic Dieting

Goal Setting: Weight Loss, Maintenance, and Muscle Gain

Setting clear goals is essential in cyclic nutrition, as it shapes the type and frequency of high- and low-carb days, as well as overall calorie intake.

- **Adapting Cyclic Nutrition to Fit Specific Goals**
  - **Weight Loss**: In cyclic nutrition for weight loss, the focus is on creating a slight calorie deficit through a higher proportion of low-carb days. By lowering carbohydrates on rest or low-activity days, the body is encouraged to use stored fat for energy. High-carb days are incorporated to prevent metabolic slowdown, provide energy for workouts, and reduce feelings of restriction.

- **Maintenance**: For those aiming to maintain their weight, cyclic nutrition can provide flexibility while stabilizing energy levels. Maintenance cycles often include an even balance of high- and low-carb days, with calories and macronutrients adjusted to meet but not exceed daily energy needs. This approach maintains muscle and energy without significant fat loss or gain.

- **Muscle Gain**: When focusing on muscle growth, cyclic nutrition includes more high-carb days to support anabolic processes (muscle building) and fuel high-intensity workouts. By incorporating high-carb days around training sessions, the body has ample glycogen for energy, aiding in muscle preservation and recovery.

Calculating Caloric and Macronutrient Needs

Understanding caloric needs and macronutrient distribution is key to creating an effective cyclic nutrition plan. This section introduces tools and methods to calculate daily energy requirements and set macronutrient targets for different days in the cycle.

- **Tools and Methods for Calculating Daily Requirements**
    - **Basal Metabolic Rate (BMR)**: The BMR represents the calories the body needs to maintain basic functions at rest. Readers are encouraged to calculate their BMR as a foundation for determining total daily energy expenditure (TDEE).

- o **Total Daily Energy Expenditure (TDEE)**: By accounting for physical activity, TDEE provides an estimate of the calories needed to maintain current weight. Online calculators, fitness apps, or manual calculations using BMR and activity multipliers can be used to find TDEE.

- **Adjusting Intake for Weight Loss or Muscle Gain**
  - o **Caloric Deficit for Weight Loss**: For weight loss, a small caloric deficit (10-20% below TDEE) is recommended to encourage fat loss while preserving muscle. This deficit can be achieved by increasing low-carb days while keeping protein intake high to support muscle maintenance.

- o **Caloric Surplus for Muscle Gain**: For muscle growth, a caloric surplus (5-10% above TDEE) is added. The surplus comes primarily from carbohydrates on high-carb days, providing the energy needed for muscle synthesis and recovery. Protein intake is also emphasized to aid in tissue repair.

- o **Macronutrient Ratios for Cyclic Nutrition**: This section explains general guidelines for macronutrient ratios on high- and low-carb days:

  - **High-Carb Days**: 50-60% carbs, 25-30% protein, 15-25% fats

  - **Low-Carb Days**: 10-20% carbs, 40-50% protein, 30-40% fats These ratios are intended as starting points, with readers encouraged to adjust based on their goals and personal energy needs.

Cycle Examples (7-Day, 14-Day Plans)

Providing sample cycles offers readers a clear starting point for putting cyclic nutrition into practice. These examples demonstrate how to schedule high- and low-carb days depending on the chosen goal and activity levels.

- **7-Day Cycle Example for Weight Loss**
  - **Structure**: 5 low-carb days, 2 high-carb days
  - **Schedule**: Low-carb days on rest or low-intensity activity days, with high-carb days before or on days with intense workouts.
  - **Expected Effects**: This cycle maximizes fat-burning potential on

low-carb days while strategically timing high-carb days for metabolic support and energy.

- **Sample Week**:
    - **Monday**: Low-carb (rest day)
    - **Tuesday**: Low-carb (light activity)
    - **Wednesday**: High-carb (strength training)
    - **Thursday**: Low-carb (cardio)
    - **Friday**: Low-carb (rest day)
    - **Saturday**: High-carb (strength training)
    - **Sunday**: Low-carb (rest)
- **7-Day Cycle Example for Muscle Gain**
    - **Structure**: 3 high-carb days, 4 low-carb days
    - **Schedule**: High-carb days are centered around intense training days to support energy and recovery.

- **Expected Effects**: This cycle supports muscle growth by replenishing glycogen and providing nutrients for anabolic processes on training days, while low-carb days prevent excessive fat gain.
- **Sample Week**:
    - **Monday**: High-carb (strength training)
    - **Tuesday**: Low-carb (light activity)
    - **Wednesday**: Low-carb (cardio)
    - **Thursday**: High-carb (strength training)
    - **Friday**: Low-carb (rest)
    - **Saturday**: High-carb (strength training)
    - **Sunday**: Low-carb (rest)

- **14-Day Cycle Example for Maintenance**
  - **Structure**: Alternating high- and low-carb days every 2-3 days
  - **Schedule**: High-carb days are used on days with moderate or intense workouts, with low-carb days following for recovery and balance.
  - **Expected Effects**: This cycle maintains energy and body composition, supporting stable glycogen levels and consistent metabolic function.
  - **Sample 2-Week Plan**:
    - **Days 1-3**: Low-carb (rest/light activity)
    - **Days 4-5**: High-carb (strength training)
    - **Days 6-7**: Low-carb (rest/cardio)
    - **Days 8-9**: High-carb (strength training)

- **Days 10-12**: Low-carb (rest/light activity)
- **Days 13-14**: High-carb (strength training/cardio)

Each example provides insight into the effects of cycling on **energy levels, mood, and performance**. High-carb days tend to improve energy and mental clarity, especially before intense workouts, while low-carb days promote fat-burning and metabolic efficiency. These effects can be fine-tuned to suit individual schedules and workout preferences.

Chapter 3

High-Carbohydrate Days

The Importance of Carbohydrates

Carbohydrates are essential for providing energy, supporting recovery, and regulating important hormones. This section breaks down the science behind why carbs are vital, especially on high-carb days in a cyclic nutrition plan.

- **Role of Carbohydrates in Energy Production**

  Carbohydrates are the body's primary fuel source. They're broken down into glucose, which fuels brain function, physical activity, and overall metabolic processes. During high-intensity workouts, glycogen (stored glucose) is essential, allowing for peak performance and endurance. High-carb days restore glycogen levels, giving the body ample energy for workouts and everyday tasks.

Recovery and Muscle Replenishment

Carbs are also key for post-workout recovery. They stimulate insulin production, which helps transport glucose and amino acids into muscle cells. This process speeds up muscle repair and prepares the body for future exercise sessions. On high-carb days, increasing carb intake post-workout helps restore glycogen and promotes quicker recovery.

- **Hormone Regulation and Mental Well-Being**

Carbohydrate intake impacts hormones like leptin and serotonin. Leptin, a hormone associated with hunger and energy balance, increases with higher carb intake, helping to regulate metabolism and reduce cravings. High-carb days can also boost serotonin levels, a neurotransmitter that contributes to mood stabilization and reduces stress. By including carbs in the cycle, individuals avoid the psychological and physiological downsides of long-term carb restriction.

Planning High-Carbohydrate Days

This section guides readers on how to effectively structure high-carb days for energy and recovery.

- **Optimal Timing for Carb Intake**
    - **Pre-Workout Carbs**: Consuming carbs before a workout helps fuel performance, particularly for strength training and high-intensity exercise. Fast-digesting carbs like fruits or whole grains are ideal as they quickly elevate blood sugar levels.

o **Post-Workout Carbs**: After workouts, a combination of carbs and protein is essential for muscle recovery and replenishing glycogen stores. Carbohydrates with a moderate to high glycemic index (such as sweet potatoes or rice) are especially effective for quick glycogen replenishment.

- **Types of Carbohydrates for High-Carb Days**

Carbohydrate quality is crucial. This section outlines optimal carb sources for high-carb days, focusing on whole, nutrient-dense options:

o **Complex Carbohydrates**: Whole grains (like quinoa, brown rice, oats), legumes, and starchy vegetables (like potatoes, squash) provide sustained energy.

- o **Simple Carbohydrates**: Natural sources of simple carbs like fruits (bananas, berries, apples) offer quick energy boosts, making them suitable for pre-workout snacks.

- o **Fiber-Rich Carbs**: Carbs high in fiber, like vegetables and whole grains, stabilize blood sugar, prevent crashes, and support digestive health.

Sample Menus and Foods for High-Carb Days

To make high-carb days easy and effective, this section includes sample menus and recommended food options. These examples guide readers on what to eat throughout the day to reach their carb goals while meeting protein and fat requirements.

- **Example High-Carb Day Menu**
  This sample menu provides a balanced approach to high-carb intake, with meal timings to support energy and recovery:
  - **Breakfast**:
    - Oatmeal topped with berries, banana slices, and a handful of nuts
    - Greek yogurt on the side for added protein
  - **Mid-Morning Snack**:
    - Whole-grain toast with almond butter and apple slices
  - **Lunch**:
    - Grilled chicken or tofu bowl with brown rice, roasted sweet potatoes, mixed greens, and avocado
    - Dressing: Olive oil and lemon for healthy fats
  - **Afternoon Snack (Pre-Workout)**:

- Smoothie with a banana, mixed berries, spinach, a scoop of protein powder, and almond milk

  o **Dinner (Post-Workout)**:
    - Lean protein (salmon or chicken breast), quinoa or whole-wheat pasta, steamed broccoli, and carrots
    - Optional: A small fruit salad for dessert

- **Grocery List for High-Carb Days** This grocery list ensures readers have the essentials on hand to make high-carb days simple and satisfying. Items are categorized for easy planning:

  o **Fruits**: Bananas, apples, berries, oranges, grapes

- o **Vegetables**: Sweet potatoes, carrots, broccoli, leafy greens, bell peppers
- o **Whole Grains**: Oats, brown rice, quinoa, whole-grain pasta, whole-wheat bread
- o **Legumes**: Chickpeas, black beans, lentils
- o **Protein Sources**: Chicken breast, turkey, tofu, Greek yogurt
- o **Healthy Fats**: Avocado, nuts (almonds, walnuts), seeds, olive oil

Chapter 4

Low-Carbohydrate Days

Why Limit Carbs?

Understanding the purpose of low-carb days is essential for seeing how they support weight management, energy efficiency, and metabolic health.

- **How Reducing Carbs Affects Body Composition and Fat Loss**

  By reducing carbohydrates, the body relies on fat stores for energy, which can support fat loss. In low-carb states, insulin levels stay relatively low, which can reduce fat storage and encourage the body to use fat as fuel. Low-carb days also help manage blood sugar levels, making it easier to control hunger and prevent energy crashes.

- **Improved Insulin Sensitivity**

  Lowering carb intake improves insulin sensitivity, making the body more responsive to insulin. This is especially helpful for fat loss and metabolic health, as it can reduce cravings and improve the efficiency of glucose utilization on high-carb days. Enhanced insulin sensitivity also prevents the buildup of excess glucose, which otherwise may be stored as fat.

- **Hormone Regulation and Satiety**

Low-carb days can help balance hunger-related hormones, such as ghrelin and leptin, promoting a feeling of fullness. Additionally, a higher intake of protein and healthy fats on low-carb days contributes to longer-lasting satiety, helping prevent unnecessary snacking and overeating.

Structure of Low-Carbohydrate Days

Proper meal structuring on low-carb days is essential to maintain energy, support metabolic health, and prevent cravings. This section provides a framework for what a typical low-carb day might look like.

- **Recommended Meals and Food Combinations for Satiety and Energy**
  - **Higher Protein Intake**: Protein is essential for satiety and muscle maintenance on low-carb days. Meals should include lean protein sources like chicken, turkey, eggs, or plant-based proteins like tofu.
  - **Healthy Fats for Sustained Energy**: Healthy fats (avocado, nuts, seeds, olive oil) provide a steady energy source and help with satiety. Combining protein with fats keeps

blood sugar stable and helps reduce the likelihood of cravings.

o **Low-Carb Vegetables for Volume**: Leafy greens, cruciferous vegetables (broccoli, cauliflower), and other non-starchy vegetables add fiber, vitamins, and volume to meals, making them filling without adding significant carbs.

- **Timing of Meals and Snacks** Since energy levels can be lower on low-carb days, meal timing is essential. Spacing meals and snacks every few hours helps maintain steady energy:

  o **Breakfast**: High-protein and high-fat meal to start the day

  o **Lunch**: Balanced mix of protein, fats, and vegetables

- o **Dinner**: Similar structure to lunch, potentially with fewer calories if energy needs are lower

- o **Snacks**: Protein and fat-based options like nuts, cheese, or boiled eggs to keep hunger at bay

---

Sample Menus and Foods for Low-Carb Days

This section provides sample menus and grocery lists for easy implementation of low-carb days. With these examples, readers can see how to create a variety of satisfying, nutrient-dense meals.

- **Example Low-Carb Day Menu** This sample menu is crafted to maintain energy and support satiety on a low-carb day:

- o **Breakfast**:
  - Scrambled eggs with spinach, mushrooms, and bell peppers
  - Side of avocado and a few slices of smoked salmon
- o **Mid-Morning Snack**:
  - Handful of mixed nuts (almonds, walnuts, or macadamia nuts)
- o **Lunch**:
  - Grilled chicken or turkey breast over a salad with leafy greens, cucumbers, cherry tomatoes, and olives
  - Dressing: Olive oil and balsamic vinegar for healthy fats

- o **Afternoon Snack:**
  - Greek yogurt with chia seeds and a few raspberries
- o **Dinner:**
  - Grilled salmon or tofu with steamed asparagus, sautéed zucchini, and a drizzle of olive oil
  - Optional side: Small portion of cauliflower rice

Each meal is designed to be high in protein and healthy fats, with an emphasis on vegetables to add fiber and nutrients without adding excess carbs.

- **Grocery List for Low-Carb Days**

This list includes staple items for low-carb days, organized by category for easy shopping:

- o **Proteins**: Chicken breast, turkey, eggs, Greek yogurt, salmon, tofu
  - o **Vegetables**: Leafy greens (spinach, kale), cruciferous veggies (broccoli, cauliflower), zucchini, bell peppers, mushrooms, asparagus
  - o **Fats**: Avocado, olive oil, nuts (almonds, walnuts), chia seeds
  - o **Low-Carb Fruits**: Berries (strawberries, raspberries) in moderation for snacks

- **Meal Prep Tips for Low-Carb Days**
  - o **Batch Cook Proteins**: Grilling or baking chicken, turkey, or tofu at the start of the week makes it easy to add protein to meals.
  - o **Pre-Chop Vegetables**: Washing and chopping vegetables in advance makes meal assembly quick and

straightforward, especially for salads and stir-fries.

- o **Use Mason Jars for Snacks**: Portion out nuts or yogurt in mason jars or reusable containers for grab-and-go snacks, making it easier to control portions and reduce carb intake.

Chapter 5

Protein and Fat in Cyclic Dieting

The Role of Protein in Muscle Preservation and Recovery

Protein is essential for muscle health, especially in a cyclic diet where energy intake varies. This section covers the importance of protein for muscle maintenance and provides strategies for optimal intake.

- **Importance of Protein for Muscle Health** Protein plays a critical role in preserving lean muscle mass, particularly on low-carb days when energy is sourced primarily from fats and protein. Adequate protein intake ensures that muscle tissue isn't broken down for energy, supporting both metabolic rate and strength.

- **Optimal Protein Sources**

Protein quality is crucial, so this section highlights the best sources of high-quality protein:

- o **Lean Meats and Poultry**: Chicken breast, turkey, and lean beef are rich in amino acids necessary for muscle repair.
- o **Fish and Seafood**: Salmon, tuna, and shrimp provide protein along with omega-3 fatty acids, supporting muscle and heart health.
- o **Plant-Based Options**: Tofu, tempeh, lentils, and quinoa are excellent choices for vegetarians, offering protein and essential nutrients.
- o **Dairy and Eggs**: Greek yogurt, cottage cheese, and eggs are nutrient-dense, easily digestible options that support recovery.

- **Protein Timing and Frequency**
  - **Post-Workout**: Consuming protein shortly after workouts accelerates recovery by delivering amino acids directly to muscles, helping repair and grow muscle fibers.
  - **Throughout the Day**: Regular protein intake every few hours (20-30 grams per meal) ensures a steady supply of amino acids, preventing muscle breakdown and supporting energy on both high- and low-carb days.

Healthy Fats for Hormone Balance

Fats are vital for hormone production, energy, and satiety. This section explains the role of healthy fats in cyclic nutrition, particularly on low-carb days, and provides guidance on choosing optimal fat sources.

- **The Role of Fats in Hormone Health** Fats are essential for synthesizing hormones, particularly sex hormones like testosterone and estrogen, which impact metabolism, energy levels, and mood. On low-carb days, a higher fat intake helps the body adjust to lower carbohydrate levels by providing an alternative energy source and supporting consistent hormone production.

- **Types of Healthy Fats**

  This part details which fats to focus on and why they matter:

  - **Monounsaturated Fats**: Found in avocados, olive oil, and nuts, these fats are heart-healthy and help regulate blood sugar levels.

- **Polyunsaturated Fats**: Sources like fatty fish, chia seeds, and walnuts are high in omega-3 fatty acids, reducing inflammation and aiding in recovery.
  - **Saturated Fats** (in moderation): Healthy sources like coconut oil and grass-fed butter can be included to provide stable energy, especially on low-carb days, without excessive carb intake.

- **Incorporating Fats into Meals**

  Readers learn to balance fat intake throughout the day by combining them with protein for greater satiety:

  - **Breakfast**: Adding avocado or nuts to a high-protein meal helps curb hunger.

o **Snacks**: Nuts, seeds, or cheese provide easy, healthy fat options.

o **Cooking Oils**: Using olive oil or coconut oil for cooking delivers fats with additional health benefits, enhancing both flavor and nutrient density.

Balancing Protein and Fat Intake Across the Cycle

Achieving the right balance of protein and fats is key to maximizing the benefits of cyclic nutrition. This section offers practical tips for maintaining an effective protein-to-fat ratio on both high- and low-carb days.

- **Finding Your Ideal Ratios**

  The right balance of protein and fat varies depending on individual goals, activity levels, and metabolic needs. This section outlines general guidelines for protein and fat ratios across the cycle:

- o **High-Carb Days**: With higher carbs, protein intake remains steady, while fat intake may be slightly lower to prevent excess caloric intake. Protein should be prioritized for muscle repair and recovery.

- o **Low-Carb Days**: Fat intake rises to compensate for lower carbs, ensuring energy needs are met and satiety is maintained. Protein remains consistent to support muscle maintenance.

- **Practical Tips for Balancing Intake**
  - o **Meal Prep and Planning**: Preparing protein sources (like grilled chicken or tofu) and healthy fats (like

portioned nuts or avocados) in advance makes it easy to maintain the correct ratios across the cycle.

- o **Portion Control**: Balancing protein and fat portions helps prevent overeating, especially when calorie intake is lower. Using measuring tools (like food scales or measuring cups) can simplify portion control.

- o **Tracking Nutrient Intake**: Using a food tracking app or journal helps readers stay aware of their protein and fat ratios, supporting accountability and helping them adjust based on how they feel and progress.

Chapter 6

Lifestyle and Activity

Training on High vs. Low Carbohydrate Days

Properly aligning workouts with high- and low-carb days helps improve energy, performance, and recovery. This section provides guidance on choosing the best type of exercise for each day to maximize results.

- **High-Carbohydrate Days**

  On high-carb days, glycogen stores are replenished, providing the energy needed for intense workouts. Ideal training options for these days include:

  - **Strength Training**: Carb intake supports heavy lifting, enhancing muscle-building potential.
  - **High-Intensity Interval Training (HIIT)**: HIIT relies on glycogen stores, so these workouts are best

suited for high-carb days when energy availability is higher.

- o **Endurance Workouts**: Carbs provide sustained energy, making them essential for long runs, cycling, or other endurance exercises.

- **Low-Carbohydrate Days**

Low-carb days are better suited for lower-intensity activities, which don't demand as much glycogen. Recommended activities include:

- o **Steady-State Cardio**: Walking, cycling, or light jogging are good low-intensity options, relying less on glycogen and more on fat stores for fuel.
- o **Mobility and Flexibility Training**: Stretching, yoga, and other mobility-

focused sessions enhance recovery and reduce stress on the body.

- **Light Resistance Training**: If desired, light resistance or bodyweight exercises can help maintain muscle activation without exhausting glycogen stores.

Rest Days and Recovery Nutrition

Rest days are critical for recovery, allowing muscles to repair and grow while replenishing energy reserves. Nutrition on these days should focus on supporting these recovery processes.

- **Optimizing Protein and Fat Intake**

   On rest days, protein intake remains high to support muscle repair and prevent muscle breakdown. Since energy demands are lower, fats can replace carbohydrates as the primary energy source, helping maintain satiety and provide steady energy:

- **Protein for Muscle Repair**: Including sources like eggs, fish, and legumes helps repair muscle fibers and reduce muscle soreness.

- **Fats for Steady Energy**: Healthy fats from avocado, nuts, and seeds keep energy levels balanced and aid in hormone synthesis, crucial for recovery.

- **Carbohydrates for Glycogen Replenishment (as Needed)**

A small amount of carbohydrates may be included to support glycogen replenishment if training is particularly intense. Rest-day carb intake can be lower than training days, but maintaining some carbs can enhance recovery and prepare the body for upcoming workouts.

- **Hydration and Electrolytes**

Hydration supports muscle recovery, digestion, and energy levels. Including electrolytes, especially after intense exercise days, can help prevent dehydration and support muscle function.

Sleep and Stress Management in Cyclic Nutrition

Sleep and stress are essential components of cyclic nutrition, impacting recovery, energy levels, and hormone balance. This section emphasizes the importance of managing these factors to support physical and mental well-being.

- **The Importance of Sleep for Hormonal Balance**

Sleep affects hormones like cortisol, insulin, and growth hormone, all of which influence fat loss, muscle gain, and energy levels. Aiming for 7-9 hours of quality sleep supports these hormonal functions:

  o **Cortisol Reduction**: Lack of sleep increases cortisol, the body's primary stress hormone, which can hinder fat loss and lead to cravings.

  o **Growth Hormone and Muscle Repair**: Growth hormone peaks during deep sleep stages, supporting muscle recovery and repair.

- **Stress Management for Optimal Nutrition Results**

Chronic stress disrupts hormone balance, increasing cortisol, which can impact appetite, fat storage, and energy. This section offers stress-management techniques:

  - **Mindfulness and Meditation**: Practicing mindfulness or meditation can reduce stress, improve focus, and enhance mental clarity, helping individuals stay on track with their nutrition goals.

  - **Physical Activity for Stress Relief**: Light activities like walking, stretching, or yoga reduce stress without overtaxing the body, making them ideal complements to a cyclic nutrition plan.

o **Establishing a Wind-Down Routine**: Avoiding screen time before bed, using relaxation techniques, or keeping a gratitude journal can lower stress and improve sleep quality.

Chapter 7

Tracking and Adjusting Your Progress

Measuring Success (Beyond the Scale)

While weight loss is often a primary goal, the scale isn't always the best indicator of success. This section highlights alternative ways to measure progress that provide a more complete picture of health and fitness.

- **Body Measurements**

  Regular measurements of the waist, hips, arms, and thighs can reveal fat loss or muscle gain that the scale might not reflect. Progress photos are also useful for visual comparison over time.

- **Energy Levels and Mood**

  Tracking daily energy levels and mood can provide insight into how well your body is adapting to cyclic nutrition. High energy, good mental clarity, and stable moods suggest a well-adjusted cycle, while low energy or irritability might indicate a need for adjustment.

- **Performance Metrics**

  Noticing changes in performance during workouts, such as lifting heavier weights, completing more reps, or feeling less fatigued, can signal positive adaptations in strength and endurance. Documenting these metrics helps track physical progress beyond appearance.

By tracking these alternative metrics, readers can better gauge the effectiveness of their approach, creating a more comprehensive view of their health journey.

Common Challenges and How to Overcome Them

Navigating common obstacles is essential for maintaining progress in cyclic nutrition. This section addresses typical challenges and offers practical solutions.

- **Plateaus**

  Plateaus are common in any nutritional approach. When progress stalls, readers can:

  - **Adjust Macronutrient Ratios**: Tweaking carb or protein intake, especially around workout days, can jumpstart progress.

  - **Incorporate Different Exercises**: Changing workout intensity or duration can break through a plateau by introducing new physical demands.

- o **Implement a Deload Week**: A week of lighter workouts can allow the body to recover, which often leads to improved results once regular intensity resumes.
- **Cravings**

Dealing with cravings is crucial for long-term adherence. Strategies include:

- o **Timing High-Carb Days for Craving Control**: If cravings are intense, shifting the next high-carb day earlier can help satisfy them.
- o **High-Protein, High-Fiber Snacks**: Choosing filling snacks, like Greek yogurt with berries or nuts, can curb cravings while keeping carb intake low.
- o **Hydration and Electrolytes**: Sometimes, thirst or low electrolytes can cause cravings, so ensuring

proper hydration is a simple way to reduce them.

- **Social Situations**

Navigating meals out, gatherings, or special events while sticking to cyclic nutrition can be challenging. Solutions include:

  o **Planning High-Carb Days Around Events**: Scheduling a high-carb day for a special event allows flexibility with food choices.

  o **Smart Choices on Low-Carb Days**: When options are limited, focusing on proteins, vegetables, and salads helps keep carbs low while allowing participation in social meals.

  o **Being Transparent with Goals**: Letting friends and family know about your nutrition goals can encourage their support and make social eating easier.

When to Adjust Your Cycle

Understanding when to adjust your cycle is essential for maintaining steady progress. This section guides readers in recognizing signs that may indicate the need for a change in their approach.

- **Signs to Adjust Macronutrient Intake**
  If energy is consistently low, recovery from workouts is poor, or cravings are persistent, adjusting the macronutrient balance may help:
  - **Increase Carbs for Energy or Recovery**: If low energy affects workouts, adding an extra high-carb day or increasing carbs on workout

days can improve performance and recovery.

  o **Reduce Carbs if Progress Slows**: If fat loss stalls, readers can try shortening high-carb phases or reducing carb intake on low-carb days to create a greater caloric deficit.

- **Listening to Physical and Mental Cues** Tuning into how the body feels can provide valuable insights into whether the cycle is working optimally:

  o **Energy and Mood Fluctuations**: If energy dips or moods fluctuate frequently, adjusting meal timing or nutrient intake can help create stability.

  o **Sleep Quality**: Poor sleep can affect metabolism and recovery. Adjusting carb intake at dinner can improve sleep quality by promoting relaxation.

- **Tailoring Based on Physical Progress**
When specific goals change (e.g., transitioning from weight loss to muscle gain), adjusting the cycle's structure can support the new objectives. For example:

  o **Transitioning from Fat Loss to Maintenance**: Increase carb intake on high-carb days and gradually adjust calories to maintain weight.

  o **Switching from Weight Maintenance to Muscle Gain**: Increase calories and carb intake slightly on both high- and low-carb days to fuel muscle growth and recovery.

Chapter 8

Advanced Cyclic Nutrition Techniques

Cyclic Nutrition for Endurance and Strength Athletes

Endurance and strength athletes have unique nutritional demands due to the intensity and duration of their training. This section explores how cyclic nutrition can be adapted to meet these high-level requirements.

- **Endurance Athletes**

  For endurance athletes (e.g., runners, cyclists), carbohydrates play a crucial role in sustaining energy during long training sessions. Strategies include:

  - **Increased High-Carb Days**: More frequent high-carb days, often coinciding with long training sessions, to optimize glycogen stores and support stamina.

- **Pre- and Post-Training Carbs**: Emphasis on carb intake before and after workouts to enhance performance and speed up recovery, potentially incorporating intra-workout nutrition for longer events.

  - **Electrolyte Balance**: Managing hydration and electrolyte intake on both high- and low-carb days to maintain energy and reduce fatigue during prolonged exercise.

- **Strength Athletes**

Strength training places high demands on muscle recovery and protein synthesis, which cyclic nutrition can support by adjusting carb and protein timing:

  - **High-Carb, High-Protein Days**: On heavy lifting days, pairing high carb with increased protein intake promotes muscle repair and growth.

- **Post-Workout Nutrition**: Prioritizing carbs and protein in post-workout meals replenishes glycogen stores, enhances muscle recovery, and supports strength gains.

- **Balancing Fat on Rest Days**: Lowering carb intake on rest days and increasing fats can aid in recovery without creating a calorie surplus.

Seasonal and Long-Term Cycling Plans

Cyclic nutrition can be adjusted across seasons or planned for the long term to support changing goals, lifestyle demands, and sustained results.

- **Seasonal Adjustments**

  Adjusting cycles seasonally allows for flexibility in training, nutrition, and lifestyle:

  - **Summer and Cutting Phases**: Emphasis on more frequent low-carb days to promote leanness, with adjustments for outdoor activities and higher hydration needs.

  - **Winter and Maintenance/Bulking Phases**: Incorporating additional high-carb days during colder months or off-season training, when the focus may shift to building muscle mass or maintaining energy stores.

- o **Spring or Pre-Event Cycles**: Short, intensive cycles (like a 4- to 6-week focus) can be used before events or vacations to achieve specific body composition goals.

- **Long-Term Nutrition Cycles** Developing long-term plans can help maintain results and avoid burnout from short-term dieting. Suggestions for sustainable cycles include:

  - o **Rotating 7-Day and 14-Day Cycles**: Alternating between shorter and longer cycles throughout the year to prevent adaptation and provide flexibility.

  - o **Maintenance Phases**: Periodic maintenance phases with balanced high- and low-carb days prevent metabolic slowdown and reduce stress from constant dieting.

- o **Incorporating Recovery Weeks**: Planned recovery weeks with moderate carb intake and reduced training intensity can enhance long-term adherence and prevent overtraining.

Experimenting with Ratios and Cycle Lengths

Every individual's body responds differently to macronutrient ratios and cycle lengths. This section provides guidance for personalizing cyclic nutrition based on individual responses and goals.

- **Adjusting Macronutrient Ratios**

  Fine-tuning carb, protein, and fat ratios can yield better results depending on individual preferences, metabolism, and energy needs:

- o **Higher Carb vs. Higher Fat Cycles**: Experimenting with a slightly higher carb or fat intake can help individuals determine which macronutrient makes them feel more energetic and satisfied.

- o **Protein Cycling**: Varying protein intake between high and low days based on training demands allows for muscle preservation while avoiding excess intake that may not be necessary on rest days.

- **Varying Cycle Lengths**

Customizing cycle lengths (e.g., 5-day, 7-day, 10-day) based on personal response allows for flexibility:

- o **Shorter Cycles**: Short cycles (3-5 days) are effective for individuals who prefer quicker transitions or have shorter goals like cutting before an event.

- **Longer Cycles**: Extended cycles (10-14 days) can help those focusing on gradual progress, muscle-building, or adapting to new training schedules.

- **Listening to Body Signals**

Emphasizing biofeedback such as energy levels, mood, and hunger cues can guide adjustments to the cycle's structure:

- **Cycle Length Adjustments**: If energy consistently dips or hunger increases, shortening or lengthening cycles can improve comfort and adherence.

- **Daily Routine Adaptations**: Adjusting meal timing and composition around work, social obligations, and training schedules creates a cycle that complements lifestyle rather than disrupts it.

Chapter 9

Recipes for Cyclic Dieting

High-Carbohydrate Day Recipes

High-carb days are essential for replenishing glycogen stores, boosting energy, and supporting recovery. These recipes focus on complex carbohydrates, lean proteins, and nutrient-dense vegetables to provide energy while avoiding excess sugars or processed ingredients.

- **Breakfasts for High-Carb Days**
  - **Overnight Oats with Berries and Almonds**

    A customizable oat base with fresh berries, almond slices, and a dash of honey for natural sweetness.

  - **Sweet Potato and Spinach Frittata**

    A baked frittata loaded with slow-digesting carbs and fiber from sweet potatoes, along with iron-rich spinach.

- **Lunches for High-Carb Days**
  - **Quinoa and Grilled Vegetable Bowl**

    A versatile, plant-based option with quinoa, grilled zucchini, bell peppers, and a light tahini dressing for added flavor.
  - **Chicken and Brown Rice Wraps**

    Lean chicken breast, brown rice, and leafy greens in a whole-wheat wrap, with hummus for a creamy, nutritious filling.

- **Dinners for High-Carb Days**
  - **Whole-Grain Pasta with Roasted Vegetables**

    High-fiber whole-grain pasta, roasted vegetables, and a light pesto sauce make a hearty yet balanced dinner.

- **Stuffed Bell Peppers with Lean Ground Turkey and Black Beans**
  Bell peppers filled with lean turkey, black beans, and brown rice, topped with a bit of cheese for flavor.

Low-Carbohydrate Day Recipes

Low-carb days are structured to promote fat-burning by minimizing carbohydrate intake. These recipes feature high-protein ingredients and healthy fats to ensure satisfaction and steady energy without the need for carbs.

- **Breakfasts for Low-Carb Days**
  - **Avocado and Smoked Salmon on Greens**
    Creamy avocado paired with smoked salmon over leafy greens, topped

with a sprinkle of sesame seeds and lemon juice.

- o **Egg Muffins with Spinach and Cheese**

  Portable egg muffins baked with spinach, mushrooms, and a small amount of cheese, ideal for meal prep.

- **Lunches for Low-Carb Days**
  - o **Grilled Chicken Caesar Salad (Dressing on the Side)**

    A classic Caesar salad with grilled chicken, leafy greens, and a low-fat dressing on the side for better portion control.

  - o **Tuna and Avocado Lettuce Wraps**

    A quick lunch using canned tuna mixed with avocado, wrapped in lettuce leaves, and seasoned with salt, pepper, and a squeeze of lime.

  - o

- **Dinners for Low-Carb Days**
  - **Zucchini Noodles with Pesto and Grilled Shrimp**

    Spiralized zucchini "noodles" with homemade pesto, topped with grilled shrimp for protein.
  - **Cauliflower Rice Stir-Fry with Tofu and Veggies**

    Cauliflower rice stir-fried with tofu, bell peppers, and broccoli for a satisfying, plant-based dinner.

Meal Prep Strategies to Simplify the Process

Meal prep is crucial for maintaining consistency with cyclic nutrition. This section provides tips and techniques to make meal prep easier and more efficient.

- **Batch Cooking Staples**
    - o **Protein Prep**: Pre-cook proteins like chicken, turkey, and tofu to have on hand for various meals throughout the week.
    - o **Grains and Starches**: Cook a batch of quinoa, rice, and potatoes for high-carb days; portion and refrigerate for easy access.
    - o **Vegetable Prep**: Wash, chop, and portion vegetables for both cooking and raw salads to save time on busy days.
- **Container Organization**
    - o Use stackable containers to portion meals for each day, labeling high- and low-carb options to stay organized.
- **Freezer-Friendly Meals**
    - o Prepare freezer-friendly options, such as soups, stews, or pre-cooked

proteins, for backup meals on busy days or low-energy weeks.

By dedicating a few hours to meal prep each week, readers can simplify their daily routines and have nutritious, ready-to-eat meals for both high- and low-carb days.

Snacks and Quick Meals for Busy Days

For those with tight schedules, snacks and quick meals are essential for staying on track. This section includes portable and easy-to-make options that align with both high- and low-carb requirements.

- **High-Carb Snack Ideas**
  - **Greek Yogurt with Honey and Granola**: A protein-rich snack with a moderate carb boost from granola and natural honey.

- o **Apple Slices with Almond Butter**: Sliced apples paired with a small amount of almond butter for a balanced, energizing snack.

- o **Hummus and Whole-Grain Crackers**: Whole-grain crackers with a side of hummus provide fiber and protein.

- **Low-Carb Snack Ideas**
  - o **Hard-Boiled Eggs with a Sprinkle of Paprika**: Easy, portable, and packed with protein for satiety.

  - o **Almonds and Cheese Cubes**: A combination of healthy fats and protein to curb hunger without adding carbs.

  - o **Veggie Sticks with Guacamole**: Crisp veggie sticks like cucumber, bell peppers, and carrots served with

guacamole for added flavor and
healthy fats.

Conclusion

As you close this book and begin to reflect on the path ahead, remember that the beauty of a cyclic diet lies in its structure and flexibility. You've learned that nutrition is far more than a rigid set of rules. It's a road that adapts with you, reflecting the natural rhythms of life, the seasons, and even your daily challenges.

With each high-carb and low-carb day, you're inviting your body to become stronger, more resilient, and attuned to its needs. These cycles are not just about weight or performance; they're about discovering what balance feels like—an intuitive, nourishing rhythm that helps you feel energized and aligned with your goals.

The food you choose, the cycles you follow, and the energy you build daily are all part of a journey to your healthiest self. Through high-energy days and low-energy days, through meal planning and workouts, you're fostering a lifestyle that flows with your natural instincts rather than against them.

With a renewed understanding of your body and its cycles, the time is yours to move forward, confidently embracing each day. Reflect on your progress, be nice to yourself when needed, and celebrate every small victory. Remember, the aim of cyclic nutrition is not perfection but progress—a sustainable path to lifelong wellness, one cycle at a time.

May this be the start of a balanced, vibrant journey to health and fulfillment. Here's to the road ahead, one day, one meal, and one cycle at a time.

The End

About Jasmin Brooks

Jasmin Brooks is passionate about helping others achieve lasting health and wellness. After her own journey through the ups and downs of weight loss, she realized that the key to success lies in sustainable habits, not quick fixes. In *Cyclic Dieting: Burn Fat and Lose Weight*, Jasmin shares her personal experiences and valuable insights, providing readers with practical tools and a clear, no-nonsense approach to reaching their fitness goals. Her mission is to save you time and frustration by delivering only the most effective strategies for lifelong health.